GOOD
INTENTIONS

A GUIDED YOGA JOURNAL
FOR A MORE MEANINGFUL PRACTICE

Jasmine Tarkeshi

ROCKRIDGE
PRESS

For general information on our other products and services or to obtain technical support, please contact our Customer Care Department within the U.S. at (866) 744-2665, or outside the U.S. at (510) 253-0500.

Rockridge Press publishes its books in a variety of electronic and print formats. Some content that appears in print may not be available in electronic books, and vice versa.

TRADEMARKS: Rockridge Press and the Rockridge Press logo are trademarks or registered trademarks of Callisto Media Inc. and/or its affiliates, in the United States and other countries, and may not be used without written permission. All other trademarks are the property of their respective owners. Rockridge Press is not associated with any product or vendor mentioned in this book.

Interior and Cover Designer: Darren Samuel
Photo Art Director/Art Manager: Janice Ackerman
Editor: Lauren Ladoceour
Production Editor: Kurt Shulenberger

Cover Photography: hsvrs/istock.
Interior Photography: ii, iii and p. 43: hsvrs/istock; v: dzika_mrowka/istock; vi, xiii and p.1: arborelza/istock; viii, ix, and p. 175: Dafinchi/istock; xii: Epitavi/istock; p. 87: marigranula/123RF; p. 131: MarcelC/istock.

ISBN: Print 978-1-64611-072-8 | eBook 978-1-64611-073-5

THIS JOURNAL BELONGS TO

_____

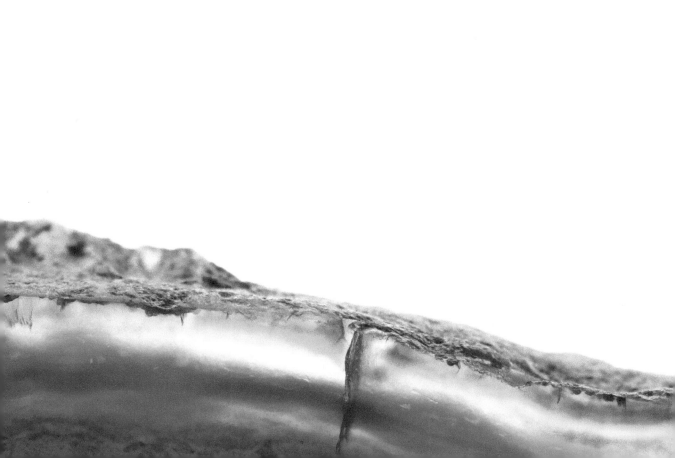

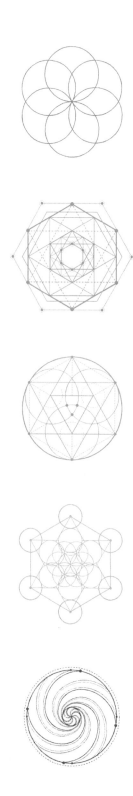

"YOGA IS THE JOURNEY OF THE SELF, THROUGH THE SELF, TO THE SELF."

—Bhagavad Gita

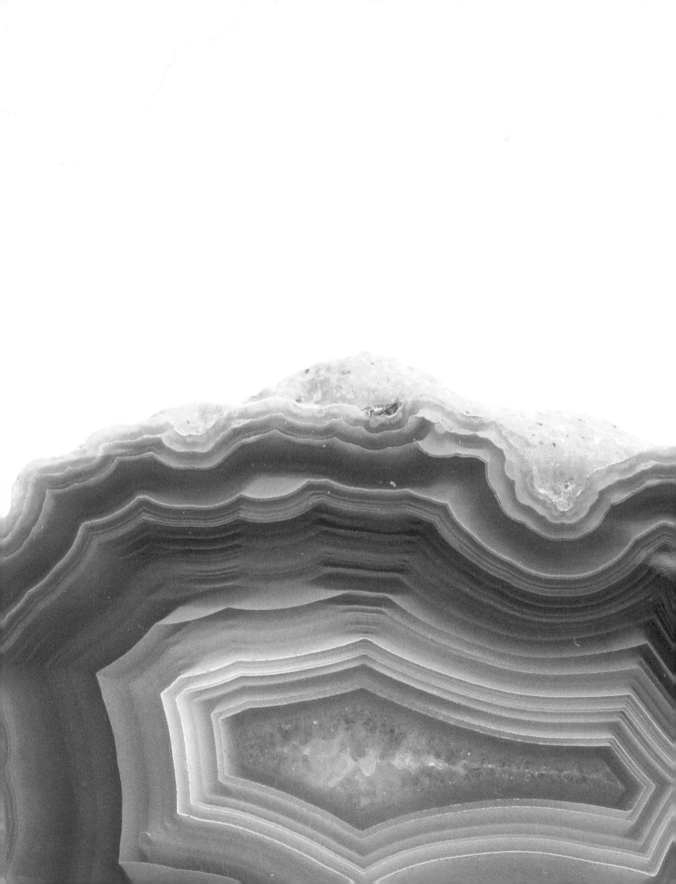

CONTENTS

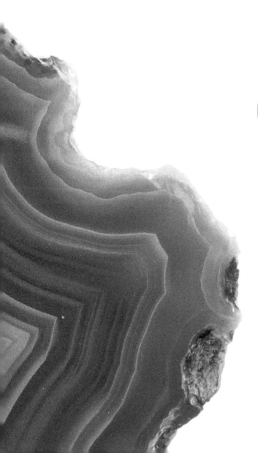

HOW TO USE THIS JOURNAL

Practicing yoga and meditation is a path to discovering your true Self, and there's no better way to take that journey than to pair practice and intention-setting with reflective journaling. I've been writing in a diary since I was a kid: pages and pages of deep questions, teenage angst, and childhood dreams for the future. When I began doing yoga as an adult, I found myself journaling once again—about the emotions that would surface during *vinyasa*; my progress with different poses; breathing and subtle body awareness; sweet meditations; and "aha" moments that would pop up during my studies of yoga's spiritual texts. Yoga is a practice of going inward, and pen and paper helped me process it all.

This journal is meant to guide and help you process your journey. Each entry begins with a short piece of yogic wisdom to digest and then suggests how to turn that teaching into a *sankalpa* (spiritual intention) for your day's practice, whether that's silent meditation, a soothing restorative sequence, energizing flow, or a *kirtan* session with your community. Teachers often ask yogis to set an intention at the start of class as a way to inspire and provide greater meaning to practice, and then to carry that intention with them throughout the day. Intentions are resolves, vows, or promises that bring yoga's teachings to life and give practice purpose. They can help you deepen your self-study by exploring yoga's philosophies and connect you to texts such as *The Yoga Sutras*, the Bhagavad Gita, and the Upanishads, which all offer uplifting wisdom. They also make yoga's 2,000-year-old roots and spiritual teachings more relevant to our modern life.

Think of intentions as prayers to weave through practice and beyond. It's nice to sit with your experience and write about it afterward. In this journal, I've included questions to help you kick-start your writing and create opportunities for growth and self-realization.

Simply select a journal entry that speaks to you in the moment, whether that means skipping around or following the book in order daily, weekly, or just every once in a while. After that, you choose how to proceed. Write freely and try not to edit yourself too much. As with yoga, there's no judgment here. The point of this journal is to open up and dig deep, letting each entry bring a new teaching and variety to your practice while supporting you on the journey to you.

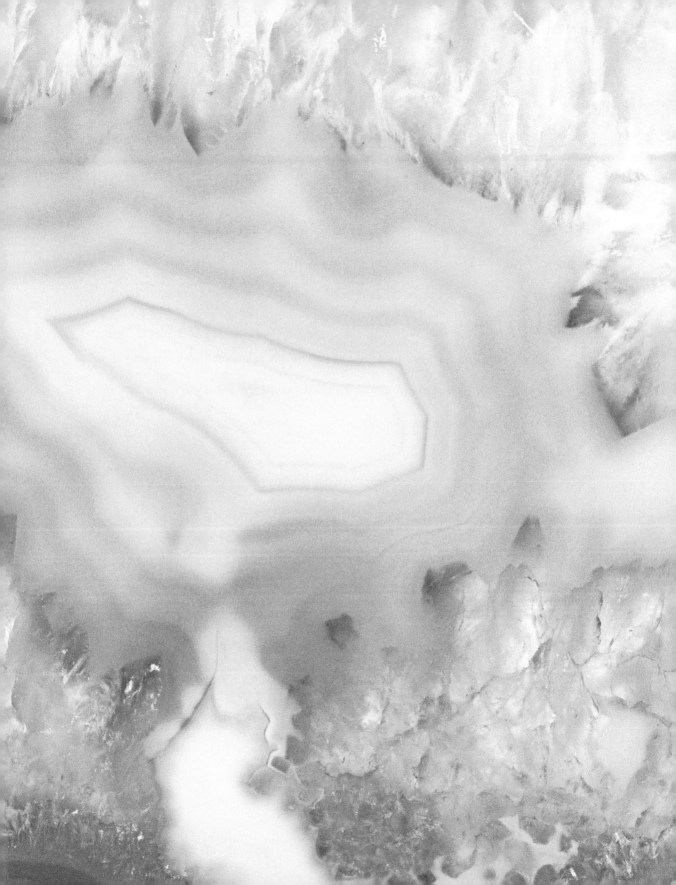

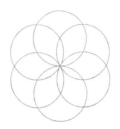

TUNE IN

NAMASTE
BOWING TO YOU

Many instructors begin and end the *asana* or meditation practice with the greeting *"namaste,"* accompanied by the hands folded at the heart in prayer and a bowing of the head.

This simple and beautiful ritual reminds us to transition from our outer ruckus to our inner refuge with reverence and gratitude. Rich with meaning, as most Sanskrit words are, it's essential to recognize the true value of "namaste" and honor its Indian roots. Derived from the root word *namah* (to bow) and *ste* (to you), namaste expresses respect as well as worship. In India this is an egalitarian greeting among all, honoring the Divine, the light, and the place that is the same within each other. The expression is also a sign of respect to teachers and elders, acknowledging their wisdom.

SET AN INTENTION

Bringing the spirit of namaste beyond the yoga studio and into the streets can have a similar transformative effect on our lives. Though we don't greet people with namaste if we aren't of Indian descent, being intentional in addressing and respecting others as our equals is a beautiful sentiment to live by, and brings the true meaning of this sacred word to life.

Namaste is more than acknowledging just the light in others; it's also about honoring the darkness and the past. This links our own experience to that of others; certainly these experiences are not the same, but they unify and bind us to each other's happiness and suffering.

Simply beginning and ending your practice or day by saying "thank you" is a profound and transformative ritual.

JOURNAL

Do I see all beings as equal? What are some of my biases? How can I live with more reverence toward others? What would it be like to bow and see the Divine in others? Can I see the light in those I admire as a reflection of my goodness?

_____

_____

_____

_____

_____

_____

_____

_____

_____

_____

_____

_____

_____

SVADYAYA
TUNE UP, TUNE IN

Our journey inward to the Self starts with tuning in to the body. In yoga philosophy, the mind and body are intrinsically linked. Balancing these two seemingly opposite qualities awakens, among other things, mindfulness and compassion. You awaken these traits first by committing to staying attentive to whatever arises, whether it's a physical sensation in the body or even your mind's reaction to an asana you may fear; and second by choosing to remain open to the experience.

Stiram Sukham Asanam, from the sage Patanjali's *The Yoga Sutras*, roughly translates to "the postures should be steady (*stira*) yet relaxed (*sukha*)." To practice this, imagine you're a musician tuning an instrument. If the instrument's strings are too tight, the strings will break; if they are too loose, no sound comes out. Being mindful of your body's movement in a yoga class is like reading sheet music, listening to each note as it's played and hearing how it affects the whole through self-study, or, in Sanskrit, *svadyaya*.

SET AN INTENTION

By becoming aware of the ping-ponging of our minds and the inner battle this causes, we can move through life's inevitable ups and downs with more balance. Every time you take your meditation seat or come into a yoga pose, you are given the opportunity to discern where you drift from the practice of Stiram Sukham Asanam. This drifting might manifest in you becoming too rigid or too passive, too tight or too loose, or in examining how you can create more equanimity in your body and mind.

As you practice, notice if you are mindlessly going through the motions or aggressively forcing your way through the experience. Remember that each extreme needs its opposite to create a balanced state of mind, and invite it in.

JOURNAL

What extremes do I fall into during my practice and my daily life and what are their effects on my mind? List where you succumb to any black-or-white thinking or extreme eating, sleeping, working, or exercising.

_____

_____

_____

_____

_____

_____

_____

_____

_____

_____

_____

PRATYAHARA
SERENADE THE SOUL

The Bhagavad Gita, the sacred Hindu and yogic text, is an allegory for the spiritual battles we fight on our quest for *samadhi* (total bliss). In the story, rife with beautiful metaphors, the self-mastery of tuning in and merging with the Self is symbolized as a rider on a chariot driven by five reined horses guided by a charioteer.

The chariot represents our body; the five horses, our senses; the reins, our mind; the charioteer, our intellect; the rider, our soul. This metaphor illustrates the goal of mastering our senses, instead of being mastered by them. Our five senses of sight, smell, taste, touch, and sound pull us outward as each horse bolts in a different direction to satisfy its desire. This causes our endless grasping for external happiness, which ultimately leads to our suffering.

We can serenade and redirect the senses toward the soul, like a snake charmer hypnotizing a serpent with his flute. This withdrawal of the senses toward the Self is *pratyahara*, the fifth of the eight limbs of yoga. The first four limbs, which include ethical guidelines of living, along with asana and *pranayama* (yogic breathing), are our external practices, and the last three limbs, which include working with our mind and merging with the Self, are internal. Pratyahara is known as the bridge between external and internal yoga.

SET AN INTENTION

As you practice, make a vow to leave the external world behind and dive inward toward the Self. Turn off your gadgets. Find true presence by feeling the sensations in your body, listening to your breath, and turning your *drishti*, or gaze, inward. Through this practice you might taste the flavor, or *rasa*, of each pose and the sweetness experienced in *Savasana*, known as *amrita*, or nectar of bliss.

JOURNAL

What are times I've been completely present and content through a sensory experience? (Perhaps watching a sunset, listening to the ocean, feeling the breeze or rain against my skin, or smelling the fragrance of flowers.) How can I use mindfulness through my senses to surrender to the bliss within?

_____

_____

_____

_____

_____

_____

_____

_____

_____

_____

_____

PRANAYAMA
A FAST CONNECTION

Perhaps the quickest way to tune in and become more connected with oneself is through the breath. This powerful tool is with us wherever we are: It helps us tap into our current state of mind, and frees us from stress and anxiety that can take over, by calming the nervous system and grounding the mind.

Although there are many *pranayama* (yogic breathing) practices, simply regulating thoughts and emotions through slow, even breath cycles can quiet the mind and anchor you, bringing you back to yourself. In this way, you can literally tune in to your true Self. Rather than seeking freedom from the challenges of everyday life, you can find freedom within them. And it starts with the breath.

SET AN INTENTION

Begin your practice with a few moments of sitting and slowing down your breath, creating a four-beat rhythm by counting the length of your inhales and exhales. Make sure your posture is alert and relaxed and place your hands on your belly to connect with the rise and fall of each breath. After a few cycles, find *ujjayi* breath, or "ocean breath," by gently constricting the back of your throat to make your breath more audible and oceanic.

The breath allows us to become more attentive to the messages our bodies and minds are trying to send us. Simply setting an intention to listen in to your practice can allow you to move and live in tune with who you are in the present moment, rather than being pulled into the past or future.

JOURNAL

Do you pay attention to your breath? List words or concepts you associate with "breathe." Does focusing on your breath help you sit with your thoughts and feelings? When do you most need to "just breathe"? Is pausing and focusing on your breath a waste of time? Your breathing has a rhythm. How can you add some gentle rhythm to your day?

_____

_____

_____

_____

_____

_____

_____

_____

_____

_____

_____

_____

_____

_____

OM
THE SOUND OF SILENCE

Most yoga classes begin and end with chanting the sound "*Om*." You may have experienced the chant's calming effect on your mind, or the beauty of all the voices in the room merging as one. But what does it mean, why do we chant it, and how can we consciously invite its spiritual meaning into life and practice?

According to yoga philosophy, the entire universe originated from sound. Chanting the mantra "*Om*," translated as "the sound of the Divine," reunites us with where we come from. This simple seed sound can break the illusion of separateness, and when chanted consciously, gives us the gift of deeper connection with ourselves and others.

Although generally spelled as it sounds, Om is actually comprised of four parts: A-U-M-Silence. A is the sound of creation, U is the sound of preservation, and M is the sound of destruction, which closes with the silence of the Divine.

SET AN INTENTION

The Yoga Sutras teach that chanting *Om* with intention and reflection is necessary to receive the benefits of this mantra. It's thought that chanting *Om* contains all of the sounds that purify speech and minds—literally, brainwashing—and allows us to begin again with a clean slate, free from obstacles on our path.

Begin your practice with a meditation on the meaning of the sound. Take a few moments to tune in to your breath and begin to chant *A-U-M* either silently or aloud, painting your entire exhale with the full spectrum of sound as many times as you like. Bathe in its effects leading you to silence. You can take this with you throughout your day whenever you feel disconnected and crave a deeper experience touching on the Divine within.

JOURNAL

How do I honestly feel about chanting Om? When (if ever) do I feel one with the universe?

DOSHAS
ENERGIES TO LIVE BY

Yoga and its allied self-care practice of Ayurveda call on us to pay attention to our ever-changing selves and what makes us different. This includes our particular constitution, made up of *doshas*. Dosha energies include *kapha* (created from earth and water), *pitta* (created from water and fire), and *vata* (created from air and ether).

These three dynamic energies can change in response to our actions, the foods we eat, the time of day, the seasons, our life stage, and any other sensory inputs that we meet. Eating, practicing, and living by our unique dosha constitution keeps us living in synchronicity with our body, mind, and spirit. Understanding the differences in the doshas can help us honor our own *dharma*, or life's purpose, and celebrate the unique gifts of others.

SET AN INTENTION

A simple way to honor your ever-changing rhythms of life is to create subtle changes that align your habits with the time of day you're practicing. The philosophy is simple: To create balance, do the opposite.

The morning hours of 6:00 a.m. to 10:00 a.m. are kapha hours, where we may feel tired, with the elements of earth and water being more dominant. Instead of eating a heavy breakfast and practicing Yin or restorative yoga, try a more energetic practice, like sun salutations, and eat a breakfast of tea, lighter grains, and fruit to start your day.

Later, from 10:00 a.m. to 2:00 p.m., is pitta time, when our internal fire and the sun is at its highest: This calls for the heaviest meal of the day and a more nourishing practice. The afternoon hours of 2:00 p.m. to 6:00 p.m. invoke vata, when we may feel depleted and ready for a nap. More grounding, restorative practices should be emphasized, leading us into the quieter evening hours.

JOURNAL

Do I feel kapha by nature, more nurturing, but inclined to being tired? Or am I fiery and active, prone to skin and digestive irritation giving me a more pitta constitution? Or do I feel ungrounded, doing many things at once, with an inclination toward vata? What are a few simple changes I can make in my life to bring me into a state of health and balance?

_____

_____

_____

_____

_____

_____

_____

_____

_____

_____

_____

_____

GANESH
THE BEGINNER'S MIND

You've likely seen the beloved elephant-headed Ganesh depicted on a yoga studio wall, in statue form on an altar, or perhaps even as a figurine on a car dashboard. Famously known as the remover of obstacles and lord of new beginnings, this Hindu deity is a welcome presence in his whimsical, big-bellied form.

The Hindu myth of how Ganesh acquired his elephant head begins with his mother. Ganesh was first created by his mother, Parvati, who longed for a son while her husband, Shiva, was away. Parvati requested Ganesh to guard the entrance to their home while she took a bath. Not recognizing Shiva when he returned from his meditative wanderings, Ganesh refused to let him inside. In Shiva's divine fury at not being allowed into his own home, he chopped off Ganesh's head. Parvati was inconsolable. To make amends, Shiva replaced his son's head with that of the first animal he saw: an elephant. To teach Shiva a lesson, the other gods decreed his son was to be honored in times of new beginnings.

Rich with symbolism, the most powerful teaching in this story is that our ego is our greatest obstacle and severing it is necessary for spiritual growth.

SET AN INTENTION

As Ganesh's story illustrates, often our obstacles are blessings in disguise. Ganesh is known for placing obstacles in front of us so we may conquer them through our practice, deepening our devotion, and strengthening our minds.

As you begin your practice, see if you can identify the obstacles in your path: perhaps a fractured relationship, or a work challenge. Rather than pushing away these seemingly unwelcome visitors, see if you can honor them.

JOURNAL

Recall a past experience when a large obstacle was placed in your path that, in hindsight, you see as a blessing. What did this obstacle teach you about yourself? Perhaps you learned something about your strength or your capacity for compassion. Think about your present obstacles. What could they be teaching you?

_____

_____

_____

_____

_____

_____

_____

_____

_____

_____

_____

_____

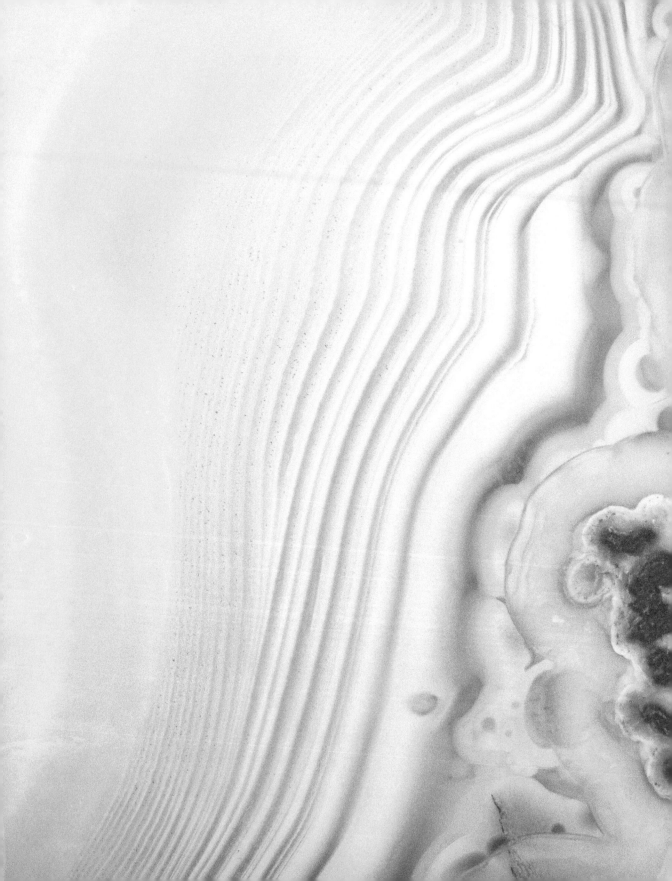

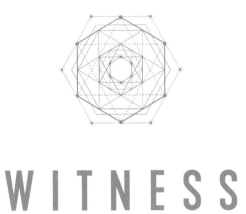

WITNESS

SAKSHI
THE WITNESS WITHIN

In yoga philosophy, tapping into our *sakshi*, or the unbiased observer within, can create true positive change in our lives. We learn in *The Yoga Sutras* that yoga is experienced by strengthening our ability to witness our thoughts and emotions—free from the bondage of our *samskaras*. Samskaras are mental imprints or habits formed from past experiences and can feel like a prison of unconscious repetitive patterns. The power to repattern our responses by pausing and discerning through the lens of our true selves is one of yoga's great gifts to daily life. This sacred moment of reflection offers the opportunity to introduce productive patterns of more conscious moving, thinking, and living.

SET AN INTENTION

Simply observe your breath—as a way to strengthen the witness within.
During practice, apply a gentle pause, or *kumbhaka*, at the height of
each inhale and the bottom of each exhale. This simple, sacred beat is a
self-check to gauge if you're moving in alignment with your higher Self
or in a knee-jerk response to the ego.

JOURNAL

Imagine you're watching a video of your life that involves a recurring situation where you react in ways you ultimately regret. Feel yourself stuck in the muck of it all and begin your journaling. Simply by naming the situation and your reaction, it can lose its power. Now, imagine widening the lens during those pauses in your breathing and call in your higher Self, the witness. Mentally time travel back to this situation. Sense how you might respond differently when your higher Self is awake. Envision how, when this situation inevitably arises again, you will introduce a more thoughtful response.

_____

_____

_____

_____

_____

_____

_____

_____

_____

_____

BHUMISPARSHA
TOUCH DOWN

You've probably seen statues of the Buddha that depict him in seated meditation with his left hand, palm upright, in his lap, and his right hand touching the earth. This hand gesture, or *mudra*, is the iconic *Bhumisparsha* (earth witness) that the Buddha took at the moment of his enlightenment. Stories tell us that right before the Buddha realized enlightenment, the demon Mara tried to distract him from his seat under the bodhi tree by tempting him with beautiful maidens. But the Buddha remained still. When temptation didn't work, Mara tried fear instead, sending terrifying armies—external ones, and also internal legions of anxieties and fear. But still, the Buddha didn't flinch. Slowly, he reached down and touched the earth. The belief is that he asked the earth itself to bear witness to his many lifetimes of perseverance and his willingness to show up no matter what was thrown his way.

SET AN INTENTION

Begin your practice with Bhumisparsha mudra by sitting tall with an alert and relaxed posture. Place your left hand on your lap facing up, symbolizing surrender, and touch the earth with your right hand, symbolizing steadfastness and wakefulness. Touching the earth is an act of humility, descending from the busy beehive of our ego, and witnessing our life as it is.

The word *humility* comes from the Latin word *humus*, the living earth. When we come back down to earth, escaping our racing thoughts and fears, we are reminded of what really matters. It is not the worries and desires that live rent-free in our minds; it is the essentials of being awake to witness and receive the beauty of the world and to give back where we can.

JOURNAL

What does humility mean to you? How can you take some time to simply observe in your daily life how you might become more awake? How can you strengthen your steadfastness in your practice and life to keep showing up no matter what?

_____

_____

_____

_____

_____

_____

_____

_____

_____

_____

_____

_____

_____

_____

VIJNANAMAYA KOSHA
WAKE THE WITNESS

According to yogic tradition, humans have five bodies or sheaths, called *koshas*, translated as "treasures." Often depicted as layers of an onion, koshas present a holistic map of five interconnected levels of being:

Annamaya kosha: The physical body

Pranamaya kosha: The physical breath and energy of anatomy

Manomaya kosha: The mental anatomy of thoughts and emotions

Vijnanamaya kosha: The wisdom sheath encompassing intellect and intuition

Anandamaya kosha: The spiritual Self

Although the health of the physical body is necessary for your well-being, it's the vijnanamaya kosha that's awakened in practice to observe thoughts, actions, and inner bliss. The witness shines a light of clarity on all aspects of the Self and governs values and ethics. When you witness your behaviors without judging them or yourself, you cultivate understanding, acceptance, and compassion. The witness is a true part of your being that, when awakened, can guide you toward wholeness and healing.

SET AN INTENTION

Awakening the witness becomes especially beneficial during challenging moments—whether on or off the yoga mat—to question what is happening within, instead of being swept away by what is triggering those challenges. Remember, you have a physical body, with thoughts and feelings, with past and present challenges, but that is not *who* you are.

Awakening your wisdom body allows you to step back from the OMGs of your human experience with wisdom and compassion, and cease identifying with what is impermanent.

To practice awakening the witness, choose a difficult yoga pose, person, or experience to concentrate on. Explore what this challenge brings up for you and observe it objectively but deeply. Step back from your actions, thoughts, and emotions to notice who is doing, who is thinking, and who is feeling the action. See if you can put a name to the thoughts, feelings, or sensations without judgment.

JOURNAL

Begin your journaling with the intention of stepping outside yourself and observing yourself and your life through an objective, unbiased lens, and write down everything you see. Look around your home and pull the lens back to see the larger picture. Then ask the big question: "Who am I? Who am I really?"

AJNA

SPY WITH YOUR THIRD EYE

In the sevenfold chakra system, known as the yogi's spiritual anatomy, the sixth chakra is called *ajna* in Sanskrit, meaning to command, to perceive, to know, or to see. Located between the eyebrows, this third eye controls intelligence, intuition, imagination, and insight. It allows you to cut through illusion and access deeper truths. Just as your two physical eyes see the outer world, the third eye is believed to connect us to intuition by revealing insights, wisdom, and meaning behind everything in life.

The energy of this chakra allows you to experience mindfulness as well as gifts of spiritual contemplation and self-reflection, seeing everything as it is from a point of witness or observer. The gift of ajna is seeing; it's the ability to receive messages and learn life lessons.

SET AN INTENTION

Take a few moments at the beginning of your practice to close your eyes and find your inner drishti: Imagine the space between your eyebrows—your third eye. Now, turn inward. Think about whatever is making you feel stuck or frozen these days (for example, a decision about a new job or a relationship), and observe the situation from a place of intuition. What's it telling you?

JOURNAL

When did you last act on your intuition? How much silence is there in your life for the whispers of your intuition to be heard? Do you look outside yourself for answers? List personal questions, such as why someone came into your life, or coincidences and experiences that contain messages. How did making mistakes enable you to learn, grow, and develop?

_____

_____

_____

_____

_____

_____

_____

_____

_____

_____

_____

_____

DHYANA
HEAVILY MEDITATED

The seventh limb of yoga, *dhyana* (or meditation), has the power to move us deeper into ourselves as we practice developing awareness of *who we are* instead of *what we do*. This is often confused with *dharana*, the sixth limb of yoga, which is the practice of one-pointed concentration on an object (like a mantra or our breath), to quiet and focus the mind. As we work to train the mind, we recognize the mental chatter and fluctuations, in Sanskrit called *chitta vritti*, which include our memories, perceptions, and imagination.

It's easy to become frustrated with our monkey minds when we sit and observe: Inner peace seems impossible to attain. You might want to push away uncomfortable thoughts and sensations rather than sit with them. But meditation is not something you're doing. Rather, it is a state of being with what *is*.

The last three limbs of yoga (dharana, dhyana, and samadhi) can't be practiced by doing; instead they are practiced by simply being, for deeper self-exploration. When you move into this deeper inner space, you go beyond the thinking mind and ego of doing, into an eternal state of being. This shift from doing to *being* happens gradually. And it isn't about just sitting there. It's a shift that will change every interaction in your daily life.

SET AN INTENTION

Your practice is not an opportunity to beat yourself up; it's a way to become more honest with yourself and realize your true Self is who you are *right now*. Discovering your true Self isn't some faraway state of perfect bliss; rather, it's the peace you will finally experience within, when you stop fighting yourself.

Set an intention to create the space to let everything in, and be with everything that arises. Take a few moments to arrive in a comfortably seated meditative posture and concentrate on your breath to rein in your mind. Then, release your focus while you practice being, not doing.

JOURNAL

What is happening inside me right now? Name thoughts, emotions, desires, and

sensations. What happens when you say something like, "let it be," and offer

unconditional acceptance to everything within you?

_____

_____

_____

_____

_____

_____

_____

_____

_____

_____

_____

_____

_____

_____

_____

_____

THE SEER
PERFECT VISION

The sage Patanjali's introductory sutras explain the power of yoga practice and how it can transform life for the better. Although in the Western world, the word *yoga* conjures the physical practice of asana, Sutra 1.2 defines it as the "constant mind chatter that distorts our perception of reality."

Yoga Sutra 1.3 states that the seer abides in itself, resting in its true nature. In other words, once we are able to still the chitta vritti through consistent practice, we can experience reality as it is rather than through the veil of our clouded minds and experiences of our past.

Reality then snaps into focus. We finally recognize our true nature, experience our connection to all that is, and realize that our lives are just as they should be! All of our practice on and off the mat is to find that undisturbed place where our mind becomes still, and clear to reflect reality, like a lake on a windless day. From this place, we are reunited with our true nature, the seer within, eliminating misconceptions about ourselves and others that lead to suffering.

SET AN INTENTION

Take a few moments at the beginning of your practice to inquire, "Who am I?"

Imagine gazing into a mirror; your eyes are mirrors to your soul. Keep gazing and asking this question, allowing your thoughts to become still. Continue investigating as all of the layers of your external identity (your age, appearance, your job, ethnicity, gender, accomplishments, and failures) peel away until there is no "me" left. What remains is your true nature: the Self that has always been and always will be present, free of judgment and with the power to see the world in its true nature.

JOURNAL

What labels and personal identifications do you put on yourself? Maybe it's your job or economic status. See if you can name some distortions of yourself or others through past experiences. How would you see yourself and the world if your vision were clear and undistorted? Write about how you would see yourself as you truly are, rather than through the clouded lens of how you should be or how you once were.

PURUSHA
THE OBSERVER WITHIN

One of the most common teachings that reappears in yogic texts from the Bhagavad Gita to *The Yoga Sutras* is Samkhya philosophy: the task of separating our spirit (*purusha*) from matter (*prakriti*).

Purusha is the witness, observer, or seer, and prakriti is nature and transient. We learn that suffering comes when we identify with temporary physical sensations and emotional responses. So, freedom from suffering hinges on detachment from prakriti: watching thoughts and emotions rather than being affected by them.

As yogis, it may seem contradictory that practice is based on detaching focus from the body. Yet the practice is intended as a lifeline to the observer within. In the Bhagavad Gita this is "the field and the Knower of the field." Understanding and contemplating this paradox illuminates practice and can lead to spiritual liberation.

SET AN INTENTION

Awakening from this dream of confusing the real with the unreal means identifying *maya*, or illusion. But our emotions *feel* so real; how could they be a dream?

In *My Stroke of Insight* by Jill Bolte Taylor, the author describes any emotional reaction as lasting only ninety seconds. After that, any remaining emotional response is because we choose to keep revisiting it. Our practice then becomes the art of "disentanglement," to become the witness, watching thoughts drift by without getting hooked on them.

To practice, begin by observing your breath and allowing yourself to be at ease. Rather than trying to quell your thoughts, allow your mind to wander. In separating ourselves from our thoughts, it's important to notice what we are thinking and develop a relationship with these thoughts. The difficulty lies in *not getting hooked on our thoughts*. Allow them to pass like clouds moving across the sky by returning to your breath.

This is one of the most transformative practices we can do to disentangle our identity from our ego Self, which is constantly grasping for external happiness, a happiness that truly *does* live within.

JOURNAL

See if you can identify your primary areas of reactive thinking. What are the repet-

itive thoughts, emotions, and storylines that take over your mind and cause anger,

anxiety, shame, or sadness? Are these fears real? Would you be truly happy if you

got "this" or "that"? What if "this" really happened? Instead of pushing these

thoughts away, try investigating what is going on inside.

_____

_____

_____

_____

_____

_____

_____

_____

_____

_____

_____

_____

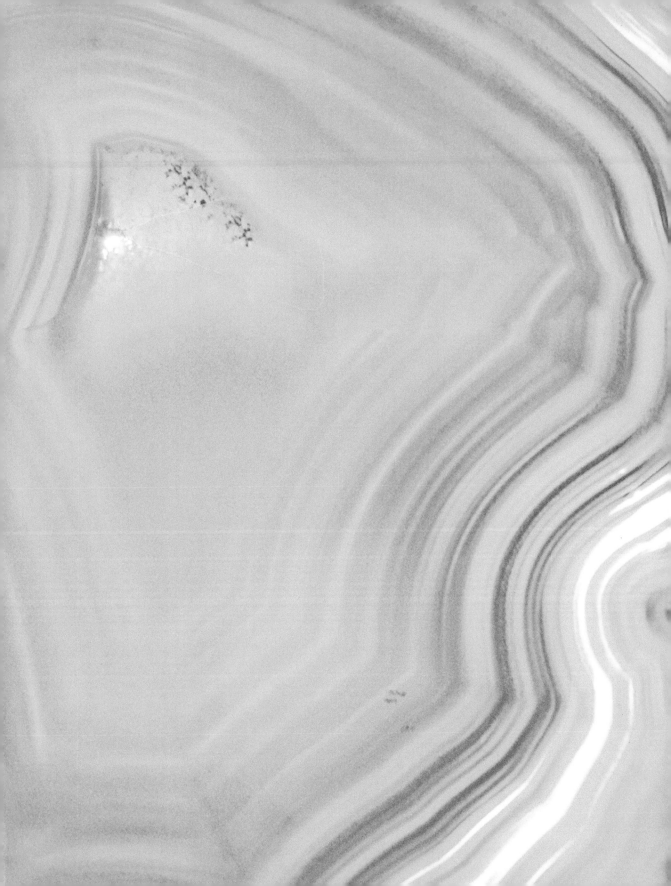

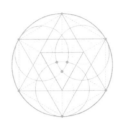

LET GO

AVIDYA
TAKING OFF THE BLINDERS

Yoga and Vedanta philosophies teach that all human suffering is attributed to the five *kleshas* (afflictions, or poison): *avidya* (ignorance), *asmita* (ego), *raga* (attachment), *dvesha* (aversion), and *abhinivesha* (fear of death). You might think of the kleshas as weeds that choke the mind and allow the conditions of suffering to root and grow.

Avidya is when we lose the essential truth of who we are, causing suffering in our lives and inviting the other four kleshas to show up.

Once we forsake our true Self, we create a false identity, the ego. Asmita is the veil that hides our true nature and causes us to become stuck. A great deal of suffering is caused by the ego's need for constant approval and control.

Raga is an undertow of fear and anxiety of losing those comforts and pleasures that we cling to. Raga creates a deep sense of insecurity within, so we hold onto our misguided life raft even tighter.

The opposite of raga is dvesha (unpleasant things that we recoil from), giving way to suffering through negative thinking, anger, or hatred.

Abhinivesha (fear of death) is the utmost attachment to life—something almost everyone experiences.

SET AN INTENTION

All of the kleshas are branches of avidya, ignorance of your true Self. Deconstructing and denouncing this mistaken identity of our false Self for our true Self is at the heart of our yoga practice.

Although pain is unavoidable, suffering is the identification with pain. In your practice, begin to focus your attention on recognizing avidya. Allow yourself to drop into its accompanying negative self-talk and resurface again and again to the experience of your true Self. Even though you may feel like you are drowning in this experience, pause and take a few breaths. When the veil lifts, those joys and pains will still come and go, but no longer define you. The reward is a fresh taste of freedom.

JOURNAL

Begin by identifying how the kleshas show up in your life. What causes you the most suffering, and which klesha does this trace back to? How does your ego identity dominate your existence? What are some of your attachments? What are some of your aversions? What do you most fear?

_____

_____

_____

_____

_____

_____

_____

_____

_____

_____

_____

_____

_____

_____

TAPAS
FAN THE FLAMES

The second chapter of *The Yoga Sutras* defines *tapas* as the transformative fire that yogis stoke in practice. In Sanskrit, *tapas* means "to burn" or "discipline." Every time you show up to practice in spite of obstacles, tapas burns away impurities of the mind and body through consistent effort. The hope is that with consistent burning, you'll free yourself from bad habits and illuminate a path to positive change.

SET AN INTENTION

Cultivating tapas is as simple as confronting poses or meditation practices that you normally avoid, letting go of ego, and building discipline (for example, dedicating ten minutes every day to meditation) and courage. Stoking tapas is a different experience for everyone; one person's inversion aversion is another's shunning of Savasana. What's important is your intention to experience the transformation that happens by burning away things that stifle spiritual growth.

JOURNAL

Write about any destructive habits you want to leave behind. What are some positive changes you can implement right now? What challenges come up when considering these changes? Are you willing to face them? What does igniting tapas mean to you?

S E V A
WISDOM IN ACTION

In a time when #yogaeverydamnday monopolizes social media feeds, asana practice can appear narcissistic with its parade of fancy poses in far-off places. This presence of yoga on social media is ironic because yogic texts like the Bhagavad Gita call upon yogis to take up *seva* (selfless service)—not selfies for look-at-me Likes. You can find seva principles across spiritual traditions, and they all require one thing: letting go of selfish desires for personal gratification and, instead, helping others simply for the sake of helping others. By dropping the focus on outcomes or rewards for doing nice things and instead aligning your actions with a higher purpose of service to all living beings, you're practicing "wisdom in action."

SET AN INTENTION

When you shift an intention from "What can I get out of this?" to "What can I give to this?" you shed any potentially selfish motives, bringing you closer to your true Self. Reflect on how you contribute to the happiness and freedom for all by beginning your practice with the intention of offering the fruits of your actions for a higher good.

JOURNAL

What are some of my best qualities? In all that I do, how can I offer myself more generously? When do I act because I am expecting something in return? How do I feel when I don't get something in return for my actions? What are some opportunities to be of service right now?

_____

_____

_____

_____

_____

_____

_____

_____

_____

_____

_____

_____

SHIVA

MAKING ROOM FOR THE NEW

Of the Hindu deities, Shiva is one of the most popular to adorn and bless Indian ashrams and Western yoga studios alike. Poised in his contradictory expressions of the disciplined, seated yogi and the ecstatic dancer, Shiva serves as a reminder that destroying what no longer serves you lets you *create* space for the new.

Nataraja, the lord of the dance, is one of Shiva's most popular forms. As Nataraja, he dances in a ring of flames, perched on a tiny demon named Apasmara-Purusha, who symbolizes ignorance, greed, inertia, and negative thoughts. This image is meant to represent cycles of creation and destruction.

SET AN INTENTION

Invoking Shiva in your practice means seeing your practice as the dance of destruction, to remove destructive habits and deeply ingrained patterns that sabotage positive change.

Begin your practice with *abhaya mudra*, the mudra of protection and courage, to create a safe and brave space to observe your negative tendencies. Lift your right hand in line with your right shoulder by bending the elbow, keeping your elbow in line with your waist. Rest your left hand palm-up on your lap.

Recall a recurring negative thought of yours and its accompanying story. Take a few breaths and silently name the thoughts or the feelings associated with them. Instead of trying to push the thoughts away, welcome or even "dance" with them until they lose their power over you.

JOURNAL

What parts of you need to be destroyed in order for a new part of you to be born?
What positive changes do you wish to create in your life? What are the "demons"
in your life that haunt you? Name them. How can they become your allies instead
of your enemies?

_____

_____

_____

_____

_____

_____

_____

_____

_____

_____

_____

VAIRAGYA
NONATTACHMENT THEORY

Whether you're honing piano, dancing, or painting skills, practicing means sticking with something for a long time. Anytime you dedicate yourself to an activity (or a person), it's easy to get attached to certain outcomes or feelings.

The yogic concept of *vairagya* means ditching any attachments that grow out of practice or dedication. For example, once the honeymoon phase is over in a new relationship and you're in the thick of the day-to-day together, issues come up: tension, disagreements, jealousies, compromises. All of these issues challenge the ego (some might say "purify" the ego), but that only happens if you stick with the relationship long enough.

In the Bhagavad Gita, Arjuna cries to Krishna, "You claim yoga is the mastering of the mind, but it seems to me to be as hard as mastering the wind." Krishna replies, "Yes, it *is* hard, but through practice and nonattachment you *will* achieve it in the end."

SET AN INTENTION

Challenge yourself to sit with an asana, meditation, or pranayama for twice as long as usual to see what thoughts and emotions come up. If you usually practice meditation for ten minutes, try twenty. If you hold Warrior II for five breaths, try ten. Continue sitting with whatever arises and practice dispassion, detaching your true Self from the thoughts, emotions, and reactions that arise. As you continually practice letting go, you'll cultivate sticking to your true Self.

JOURNAL

How do you feel about practicing dispassion? Are you willing to let go of your reactions to truly be free? Write about something you've tried to be consistent with but have given up because your emotional responses were triggered. Maybe it is your asana practice, mastering an instrument or language, or entering a relationship. What are your triggers? What if you stuck with your endeavor, despite these obstacles, by letting go of the issues that came up?

_____

_____

_____

_____

_____

_____

_____

_____

_____

_____

_____

APARIGRAHA
RENOUNCE AND REJOICE

As yogis living in a modern world, our attachment to our belongings seems to define us. Think about it: the house, that car you saved up for, or maybe a treasured family heirloom. This is why the practice of *aparigraha*, or non-hoarding and non-coveting, is an integral part of our practice.

As one of the five *yamas*, or ethical vows of yoga, aparigraha serves as a daily dose of cosmic common sense to lessen the pain in our lives that comes from equating happiness with material wealth. Our yoga practice calls on us to see this trap of pursuing material goods and do the opposite. By renouncing our material possessions, we are freed up to devote our time and energy to go after the one thing that *will* give us eternal happiness: discovering our true selves.

SET AN INTENTION

There are a lot of pauses in a yoga or meditation practice where the mind can begin to wander—and often it wanders into your to-do list: things you need to pick up at the grocery store that night, an outfit you're planning for an upcoming event, the raise you hope to ask for on Monday. At the start of your practice, make a silent vow to yourself to spend this time free of these lists. They'll likely still pop up, but when they do, make note of it and, without judgment, return to your vow.

JOURNAL

Which material possessions do you find yourself most attached to? Are there any that no longer serve you? How would it feel if they were to suddenly disappear? What would you do if you had only the bare necessities and could go anywhere and do anything you wanted?

SAVASANA
THE POWER OF RELAXATION

As stated in a popular spiritual proverb—"Let go or be dragged!"—it isn't the letting go that's so painful; it's the holding on. Corpse Pose is the yogi's physical practice of letting go of attachments and opening up to living on life's terms. When you are in Corpse Pose, you can get a taste of true *ananda*, or bliss. This is where we surrender our will and tendency to control and see the bigger picture, trusting a higher power so we can detach from outcomes.

SET AN INTENTION

Take time each day to balance any active practice with deep relaxation. Although it looks easy to just lie down and relax, Savasana can be the most challenging pose. This is your time to consciously relax your body and mind and practice letting go, rather than napping or letting your mind skip ahead to what's for dinner.

To do this, lie down on your back with a rolled-up blanket under your knees, like you're being cradled. Tense every part of your body and intentionally let go with an exhale, signaling the transition from action to stillness and relaxation. Notice any part of your body still holding tension, like your jaw, shoulders, or low belly, and allow your breath to wash the tension away. You can repeat the mantra "let" on the inhale and "go" on the exhale for a few breath cycles, trusting that everything is unfolding exactly as it should for your highest good. As you detach from the limitations in your mind, you're awakening to your true Self and the new beginnings and experiences that come with it.

JOURNAL

What is your attitude toward relaxation? Are you battling an issue in your life with

your willpower? Do you feel like you're alone or left in charge of your own destiny?

Does your identity begin and end with your job? What are some things you want

to do as your true Self? What adjectives would describe your true Self?

_____

_____

_____

_____

_____

_____

_____

_____

_____

_____

_____

_____

_____

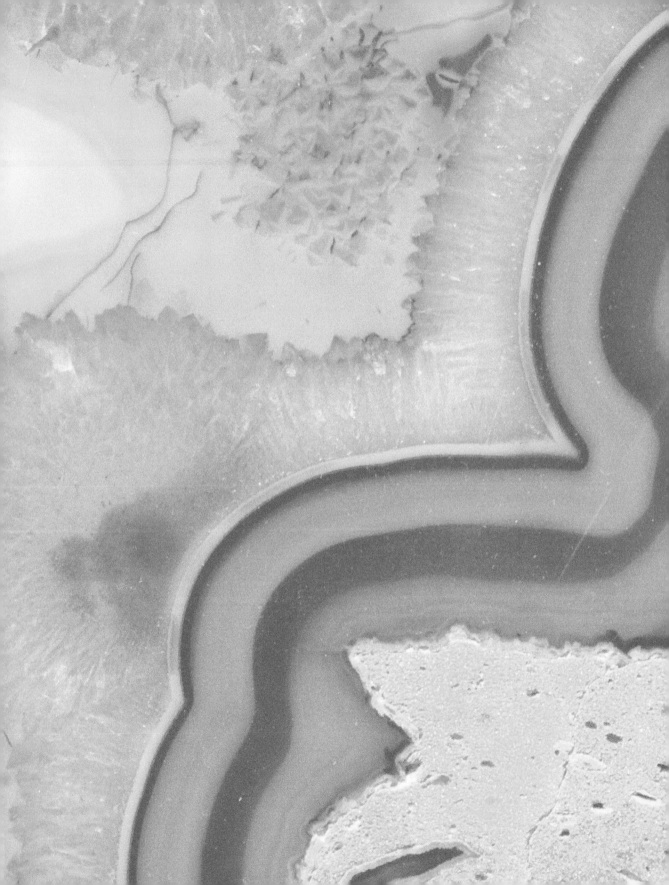

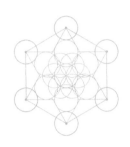

CARE

KALI

THE SELF-CARE GODDESS

Despite what your Instagram feed might indicate, life and health are not just about bubble baths and face masks. Taking care of yourself means awakening the fierce mother within that protects and guards her child from danger. This mother figure is depicted as the Hindu goddesses Kali (draped in skulls and dripping blood) and eight-armed Durga (bearing weapons and battling ferocious demons while riding a tiger), terrifying images that represent fierce acts of care, protection, and compassion in our practice.

Discipline is often perceived as punitive, but as any mother will tell you, it is served up with tough love to instill a healthier, more balanced way of living.

SET AN INTENTION

To awaken this compassionate energy in your practice, challenge your-self to commit to the practice of *saucha*, purity. As one of the *niyamas*, or "positive duties," saucha is meant to nurture good habits as a posi-tive act, not as a self-flagellating one.

As with a devoted mother, saucha encourages you to clean your home, wash your hands, bathe, eat a healthy, clean diet, and give up unhealthy habits. This fierce and loving presence is also watching over what you watch, read, think, and say.

On the mat, a disciplined practice is thought to cleanse the mind and ring out impurities from your bodily systems through sweat and the breath.

JOURNAL

What does self-care mean to you? Do you show up to your practice out of love or punishment? How do you feel about purifying your body, mind, and actions? What negative behavior is the most difficult for you to let go of? Why do you think that is?

BHAKTI
THE ROAD OF LOVE

Bhakti yoga is the path of liberation and transformation through complete devotion to the Divine. That divinity could be a deity, a spiritual principle like peace, an image of a saint, parent, child, friend, or something else entirely—whatever inspires the whole range of human emotions in you. Instead of longing to be the beloved, we choose to become the lover.

Love can transform us in ways that asana practice can't on its own. Learning to love unconditionally is a journey, and at the end of the journey is the realization that love is a form of the Divine within all of us.

SET AN INTENTION

Creating an altar or sacred space in your home can be a simple way to awaken *bhakti* in your personal practice and life. Here are some suggestions of what to include on your altar:

- Images of people, objects, or places that awaken a pure feeling of love
- Traditional statues of deities that represent spiritual qualities you wish to embody
- Art, musical lyrics, poetry, or any objects that connect you to your heart
- Fresh flowers and incense to make the altar come alive

Take a few moments to sit in front of your sacred space. Instead of closing your eyes, take time to connect with every element of your altar as your heart surges with feeling. Then make your offering with a simple personal prayer of gratitude or even a traditional Sanskrit mantra, if this connects you to your heart. The point of this practice is to be in a constant state of love and to see all beings as sacred to serve as the Divine.

JOURNAL

How can you awaken bhakti in your life? Write about the many ways to be in love—beyond the traditional societal constructs of this phrase—and write about how you might become even more loving. What are ways to practice bhakti on the mat? Write about how you can make your practice an offering of love.

_____

_____

_____

_____

_____

_____

_____

_____

_____

_____

_____

AHIMSA
FIRST DO NO HARM

Through the first yama of *ahimsa*, or nonviolence, we create an internal atmosphere of love and compassion, devoting ourselves to not causing harm to any being through word, thought, deed, or action.

Although ahimsa seems to benefit others, it is intended to commit us to our true Self, where future suffering in our lives can be avoided by what we do now.

SET AN INTENTION

Beginning your practice with an intention is a vow in itself. Begin by joining your hands at your heart in prayer to honor your commitment of nonviolence to yourself. Take a few breaths to tune in, and imagine yourself at your altar saying your sacred vows to the beloved within. You could vow to honor an injury or not push past your limits. Or you could vow to not judge yourself with negative self-talk and accept where you are in your practice.

JOURNAL

Write down your vows by listing all the ways you can lessen harm through your actions in the world. What are some ways to lessen your impact on the earth? What language can you use with others to bring more kindness into their lives? What language can you use with yourself?

_____

_____

_____

_____

_____

_____

_____

_____

_____

_____

_____

_____

_____

SAMA VRITTI
THE HEALING BREATH

Although all aspects of our yoga practice are of great value, pranayama, the fourth limb that encompasses breathing techniques, cares for all our needs. Pranayama techniques like *sama vritti* (even inhales and exhales) are a built-in tool we have at all times to quiet and focus the mind, nurture the body, regulate emotions, and live mindfully.

With each inhalation, we become aware of what we take in, and with each exhalation, what we give out. Our lungs are the forests of our bodies, giving oxygen and removing carbon dioxide. Every inhale is nourishing, and every exhale is cleansing. Our very lives can become a practice in sama vritti, taking in only what is life-giving and letting go of all that is toxic.

SET AN INTENTION

Begin by lying down with the intention to simply nurture yourself with your breath. Make sure you feel warm by perhaps placing a blanket over you. Place your hands on your belly and feel your abdomen rise and fall as you breathe in and out through your nose. This stimulates the rest-and-digest response in the body instead of fight-or-flight.

Create an evenness in the length of your inhale and exhale. After a few minutes, inhale through your nose and exhale through your mouth, releasing anything toxic from your body or mind. Where is your body holding tension? Are you holding on to anything emotionally? See if with each exhale you can release a little bit more of that tension.

Return to breathing in and out through your nose naturally and move your hands up to your heart. As you inhale, feel your heart rise up into your hands, like a swell in the ocean. As you exhale, imagine compassion pouring out to others. When you are ready, open your eyes and take a few mindful breaths before coming up to sit. Acknowledge the power of creating a loving space for yourself.

JOURNAL

What's your relationship like with your breath? Are you aware of it in your day-to-day actions? Make an effort to notice the quality of your breathing and what happens when you stop, pause, and breathe. What happens to your mind and body?

SAMADHI
KEYS TO THE HEART

In *The Yoga Sutras*, Patanjali outlines many practices to still the mind's fluctuations and preserve inner peace. Sutra 1.33 guides us to use our relationships with others to experience *samadhi*, or union with our essential selves, by cultivating keys to the heart, including *maitri* (kindness) and *karuna* (compassion).

SET AN INTENTION

To explore and awaken these qualities, begin with yourself. When we practice maitri and karuna, we start by befriending ourselves before attempting to befriend others. Self-acceptance can be challenging. But in being kind to yourself, you might discover feelings that you've been ignoring and that have subconsciously sabotaged relationships.

To begin, come to a comfortable seat and remember a time when you said or did something kind or caring. It could have been holding the door for a stranger or bringing coworkers coffee. The recognition of these simple acts of kindness are doorways to loving and being loved unconditionally.

JOURNAL

How would you like to be loved for who you are without having to do anything

different? Are you kind and compassionate with yourself when you are suffering?

What are some ways you can nurture these qualities with others?

_____

_____

_____

_____

_____

_____

_____

_____

_____

_____

_____

_____

_____

ANAHATA CHAKRA
UNCONDITIONAL LOVE

Pop culture tells us love comes from an external source, rather than it *being* the source of who we are. But the Vedic text the Upanishads reminds us, "From love we come; to love we shall return." All of our practices are meant to reunite us with where we actually come from: our original state, which is love itself.

In yogic teachings, this love resides within the fourth chakra *anahata*, meaning unstruck sound. Located within the heart and lungs, it bridges our physical body, mind, emotions, and our spiritual Self. This chakra is our source of unconditional love, relationships, compassion, forgiveness, and joy.

Although love is often deemed as being soft, it's what we need the most strength for. Our challenge is to pass the daily test of unconditional love, compassion, and forgiveness by building courage to stay open and vulnerable. We then work toward accepting our shadow side to experience self-acceptance and awaken unconditional love for others.

SET AN INTENTION

A back-bending practice is the remedy to build the physical and mental strength you need to stay open. Poses such as Camel, Cobra, Upward-Facing Dog, and Wheel create strength in our back muscles to support the openness of our chest, lungs, and shoulders. By awakening and healing the anahata chakra in our practice, we surrender to the potency of love, and the vulnerability that comes from entering into loving relationships with others.

Sit upright and draw your shoulders back to widen and lift your chest. Rub your hands together to create some heat and place them on your heart, allowing the warmth of your hands to thaw your heart. Take a few nourishing breaths into your heart and repeat some positive affirmations to yourself: "I love myself for all that I am." "I'm grateful for the unconditional love in my life—the love I receive and the love I give."

JOURNAL

Am I compassionate? Do I judge others? Am I hard on myself? Do I honor my dark side as well as my light side? How connected do I feel with others? Do I listen to my heart or mind more? Am I willing to forgive to heal past hurts?

_____

_____

_____

_____

_____

_____

_____

_____

_____

_____

_____

_____

_____

DHARMA
ANSWERING THE CALL

The Bhagavad Gita overflows with rich wisdom and poetic prose on achieving spiritual liberation. The setting is an internal battlefield where a dramatic war is ready to break out between the forces of darkness and light. At the heart of the scene is Arjuna, a warrior struggling with his duty to fight, and his reluctance to follow his own authentic calling, or *dharma* in Sanskrit. At our core, we understand there is no fiercer battle than the one we experience within.

Not living our dharma is at the core of our suffering. As the Bhagavad Gita sings, "Better to live your own dharma imperfectly than living someone else's perfectly."

Just as Arjuna fights and finally embraces his calling through the teachings of yoga, so must we embrace who we are and show up for ourselves in a way that honors our unique dharma without either comparing it or judging it based on other people's dharma. As Oscar Wilde once said, "Be yourself. Everyone else is taken."

SET AN INTENTION

Unfortunately, no one else can teach you or tell you what your purpose is: *You* have to be the one to discover it.

One way to do this is through a daily ten-minute meditation practice, to meet and accept yourself as you *are*, not by what you *do*. Through deepening this honest relationship, you'll get closer to discovering your dharma.

The more we meditate, the more we cultivate *shraddha*, or faith in destiny. This is the confidence that everything in your life has a purpose and is leading you toward your true calling.

Perhaps there is a message being repeated that you're not letting in: Allow yourself to be attentive to it. By strengthening this connection to shraddha, you'll find it becomes increasingly difficult to go back to your old life and easier to live the life that awaits you.

JOURNAL

Does your home and job reflect who you are now? Do the people you surround yourself with and your creative or leisure pursuits reflect who you are now? If not, what are some actions you can take to begin to follow your truth? List these actions and write about how they would feed your soul.

_____

_____

_____

_____

_____

_____

_____

_____

_____

_____

_____

_____

_____

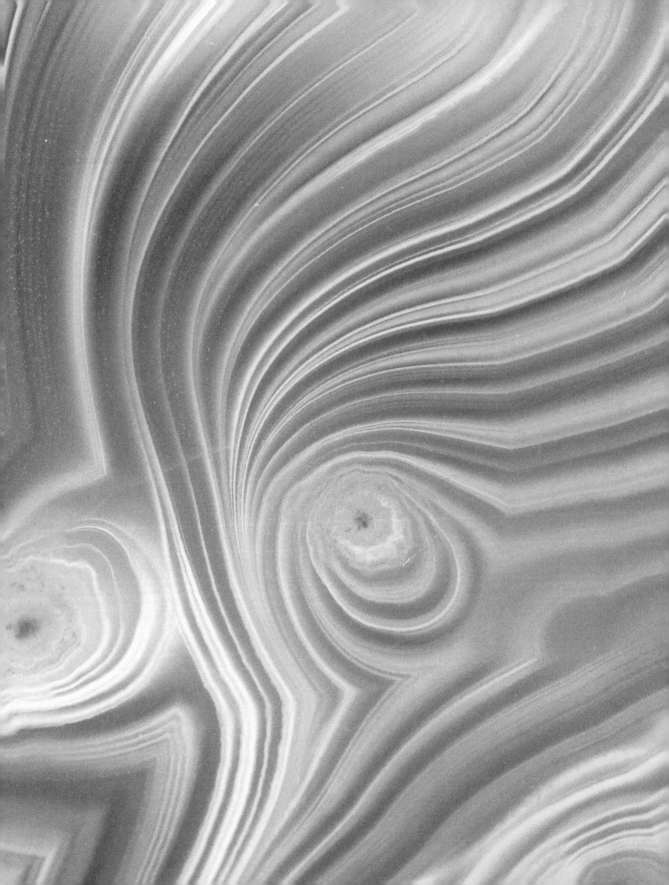

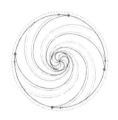

GRACE

KRIPA
OPENING TO GRACE

Kripa is a Sanskrit word meaning mercy and Divine grace. However, kripa isn't a gift from a guru or god, but rather an experience earned through effort. The experience of kripa is a catalyst for a yogi to begin the path of spiritual transformation, and the ultimate key to unlocking self-realization.

We may experience kripa during Savasana when we receive the blessings of our tapas and experience the hard-earned bliss of our effort. This grace continues to unfold as we move through the day with less struggle and more faith, feeling less shaken by the outside world and more present, spreading the blessings of our practice to others.

There are four main types of kripa:

Atma kripa: The grace of the Self

Guru kripa: The grace of the guru

Shastra kripa: The grace of the scriptures

Ishwara kripa: The grace of god

SET AN INTENTION

Contemplate an obstacle you're facing and look to the yogic teachings of *The Yoga Sutras* or Bhagavad Gita to receive shastra kripa, letting the wisdom guide you in your practice. In this way, you are approaching your practice with faith that it will lead you to grace.

Guru kripa is one of the greatest gifts of yoga. Do you currently have a trusted spiritual teacher you're devoted to? If not, set out to find one. Ask for guidance on your spiritual path and let go of your teacher when you feel called to experience grace and faith in a higher power.

JOURNAL

Begin by acknowledging grace in your life; for example, the parts of your life that are effortless or even those times when you felt blessed by the teachings of someone who impacted your life's direction. What is your relationship to the word guru? How do you feel about having a teacher? What is your relationship to the word god?

_____

_____

_____

_____

_____

_____

_____

_____

_____

_____

_____

VINYASA
MOVING WITH GRACE

Although characterized by fast-moving classes set to curated playlists, *vinyasa* is more than a flowing asana class for modern times. Various definitions of the Sanskrit word include "to place in a special way," "wise progression," and "moving with grace."

Vinyasa or vinyasa karma is a yogic approach to moving with intention and grace from start to finish. But it's not relegated to time on the mat. We can call upon this concept to do *everything* in an intentional way, from entering the yoga studio with awareness to unrolling our yoga mat with solemnity instead of a slap. The moment we reach the end of our practice is as important as the moment we begin the transition to what's next. What if you didn't check your phone for messages as soon as class ended? What if you gathered your things after Savasana with as much ceremony as flowing through Sun Salutation?

Whether you're cooking a meal or walking to work, consider each event an opportunity to be aware of thoughts, words, and actions. How you climb up a mountain is as important as how you descend it. So it is with life. In the end, it all comes down to grace.

SET AN INTENTION

Instead of approaching your practice as something to check off your to-do list, set the intention to celebrate the journey and not just the destination. Take a few moments to surrender to the flow of your breath. This intention spiritualizes your practice by connecting you to a source of peace, love, and grace.

As you begin to move, let your breath take the lead, like moving to music. With conscious breathing comes conscious moving, and your practice becomes a moving meditation. In a challenging yoga practice, intention and grace can teach you to move through life's challenges.

JOURNAL

Do you find yourself rushing or pushing through everything you do—including your yoga practice? What would it be like to slow down and move through your day without conflict or resistance? Write down a plan for your day that includes the intention to approach it as a moving meditation rather than a checklist to get through and something to survive.

ISHVARA PRANIDHANA

LIVING WITH GRACE

There is a sacred evolution when yoga shifts from being something you do to who you are. This is the transformation of becoming a yogi and leading a spiritual life. In Sanskrit, this surrender to a higher purpose or power is called *ishvara pranidhana*, knowing that what's best for us is always present and all-powerful, guiding us toward our highest potential.

SET AN INTENTION

A beautiful way to begin your practice is by lying down on your belly with your arms outstretched and palms facing up as an act of surrender. You can silently offer a personal prayer or one that resonates with you. Like planting a seed, even one line of the St. Francis prayer ("Make me an instrument of thy peace.") can transform your practice by welcoming into your life exactly what you sow.

Approach your mat as a sacred altar where each movement becomes an offering, a moving prayer. The Sun Salutation, bowing and giving thanks for the source of light, is such an offering.

JOURNAL

What do you long for? What are some ways you can give what you want? If you want more love, how can you be more loving? If you want more abundance, how can you be more generous? If you want more peace, how can you cultivate more of it in your life?

_____

_____

_____

_____

_____

_____

_____

_____

_____

_____

_____

_____

VEDANTA

ALL THAT I AM

Vedanta is a philosophy taught by the Vedas—the most ancient scriptures of India. Their fundamental teaching is that our real nature, called our *atman*, is Divine; *Brahman*, or god, exists in every being, and therefore a search for the Divine is within. Brahman is in everything, and everything is Brahman.

Swami Vivekananda, the great yogi responsible for bringing yoga to the West, said, "If a man doesn't believe in a god outside himself, he is considered an atheist, whereas Vedanta says that a man who doesn't believe in himself is the atheist."

Rather than thinking we need to be found or saved, we learn in the teachings that we are never lost. We are simply living in ignorance of our true nature.

SET AN INTENTION

Instead of approaching your practice as self-improvement, step onto your mat imagining you are already perfect, Divine, and free. Begin by silently telling yourself, "I am Divine." In this way, your practice becomes a celebration of your true Self: pure peace, joy, and love within, to be shared with the world.

JOURNAL

Write about the virtues that are already within you and in all you do. There are only two rules in this exercise: Do not stop to think, and don't cross anything out. Just let your pen keep moving as an ode to the Self. You may not be able to stop writing!

JIVANMUKTA
THE LOTUS IN THE MUD

The exquisite and fragrant lotus flower rooted in a pond's muddy waters is a beautiful symbol to inspire spiritual practice. Just like the lotus blooming from the mud with nary a drop of dirt sticking to it, we too can experience liberation *within* our own murky circumstances.

In yoga, this image expresses the teachings of *jivanmukta*, one whose belief is finding liberation not in the afterlife but in the here and now.

This mind-set transforms how we treat others, that is, with respect regardless of how they may treat us. We become humble, patient, indifferent to gain or loss, courageous, and honest, speaking clearly yet with kindness. As the exquisite lotus beautifies its own murky environment, we too can transform the environmental and political landscape through radiating kindness, peace, and courage for the welfare of all beings.

SET AN INTENTION

Begin in a seated meditative posture with the *padma* or lotus mudra. Place both hands in front of your heart with the outer edges of your little fingers and thumbs touching, and the base of your hands and wrists coming together to form a lotus flower. Spread your fingers wide while keeping your little fingers, thumbs, and wrists together. Turn your gaze and focus toward your hands, envisioning a beautiful flower, and breathe deeply as if you were inhaling the flower's fragrance.

Set the intention in your practice to tap into the grace and freedom in your movements, no matter the heaviness you may feel in your physical body or in your life overall. This intention is not meant to ignore discomfort, but instead to experience the freedom that lies within these challenges.

JOURNAL

In what ways can you be the lotus within the mud of your life? Write about the dynamics in your life that you find particularly challenging. (You may start with a relationship in which the challenge seems to be someone else's fault and all would be fine if they changed.) List ways you can shift this dynamic, through your reactions, to retain your peace of mind, despite being surrounded by the mud.

MANTRA
HAPPY AND FREE FOR ALL

Although yoga philosophy is as vast as the sky, nothing summarizes the power of our practice more than the Sanskrit mantra, "*Lokha Samastha Sukhino Bhavantu.*" This is an ancient Hindu prayer that's commonly chanted in yoga classes around the world and translates to: "May all beings everywhere be happy and free." Though most of us begin our practice with the purpose of a quiet mind and healthy body, with consistent practice we soon become aware of how our practice and mindful living can benefit all.

Generally, we associate prayer with making a wish list for ourselves, but as yogis, our mind becomes more expansive when we pray for the welfare of all beings: humans, animals, even plants. Through such a prayer, we slowly transcend our egocentric concepts of Self to identify with all of creation, recognizing creation's true nature to be one with our own. As we too are part of the universe, we also benefit from the blessings of the prayer.

The greatest blessing of this mantra is that it's not merely a recitation, but a living, breathing prayer of action that we bring to life, as it continues with "and may the thoughts, words, deeds, and actions of my own life contribute in some way to that happiness and to that freedom for all."

SET AN INTENTION

Take a few moments with your hands at your heart in prayer to tune in to your breath. Consciously experience your *prana*, your life force, and its connection to the prana of all beings. Imagine the world's people, animals, insects, and plants breathing the same breath, and tap into the sanctity of each and every life. If you feel comfortable chanting in Sanskrit, recite the mantra slowly, feeling the virtue of each word. Otherwise, repeat it in English.

Through your asana practice, you express your interconnectedness with *all* life by taking on the shapes of birds, cows, trees, mountains, the sun, and the moon. This reminds you to identify with all beings and that every action affects the whole. Through asana, your whole practice becomes a prayer.

JOURNAL

How can you take your practice and prayer off the mat and into the streets?

What are some actionable ways you can directly lessen the suffering in the world?

Are there organizations you feel aligned with that you can support? How do you

align your simple everyday actions with bringing more happiness and freedom to

the world?

ATHA
EXPERIENCE THE NOW

Atha Yoganushasanam: "Now begins the practice of Yoga."

This is the dramatic first *sutra*, or thread, of the sage Patanjali's 2,000-year-old yoga guidebook, *The Yoga Sutras. Atha,* meaning "now," is symbolic of an auspicious beginning, and *iti,* "that is all," indicates the end.

This relationship is expanded on in the fourth chapter of the Sutras titled "*Kaivalya Pada,*" which ends with the word *iti.* This chapter summarizes the yogi's outlook on life. *Kaivalya* means emancipation and even solitude, indicating wholeness as the goal of yoga.

"Just as when the clouds disappear, the sky clears and the sun shines brilliantly, the Yogi is crowned with the wisdom of living in the eternal and internal Now. The entire Now is Divine and so is the yogi, a fulfilled soul, living in benevolent freedom and beatitude, alone and complete. Besides this search for the soul, there is nothing."

SET AN INTENTION

Instead of beginning your practice as a means to an end, begin with chanting the word *atha* (pronounced ah-tah). Atha whispers a reminder that all yoga teachings emerge from and lead you back to the now, the only moment when *yoga* exists. Allow it to grab your attention at the moment you depart from your everyday identity to assume a new role as a yogi.

Say the chant silently in Sanskrit or English and notice if it draws you into the present. Close your eyes, lengthen your spine, and draw out each breath. When you exhale, think "now" and feel the present moment.

JOURNAL

What is your relationship to the word now? *Write about your life in this moment. What are some ways to make peace with your life right* now *as it is, as the only moment there is? List all the ways you can become more present and, therefore, whole, peaceful, and free, as if nothing is missing.*

_____

_____

_____

_____

_____

_____

_____

_____

_____

_____

_____

_____

_____

ABOUT THE AUTHOR

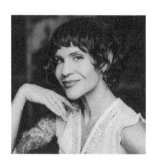 **Jasmine Tarkeshi** is the cofounder and director of Laughing Lotus Yoga Centers in San Francisco and New York City and is the author of the *Yoga Body and Mind Handbook*.

She teaches her signature Lotus Flow style of yoga in studios and online at Yoga Anytime, and leads guided meditations and teacher trainings across the globe. A respected yoga teacher for more than twenty years, Jasmine has been featured in the pages of *Yoga Journal, Elle, The New York Times*, and the *San Francisco Chronicle*. She lives in San Francisco, California, with her daughter, Indigo.